Superfoods KALE

21 Healthy and Easy Recipes to Nourish the Mind, Body and Soul.

TABLE OF CONTENTS

INTRODUCTION

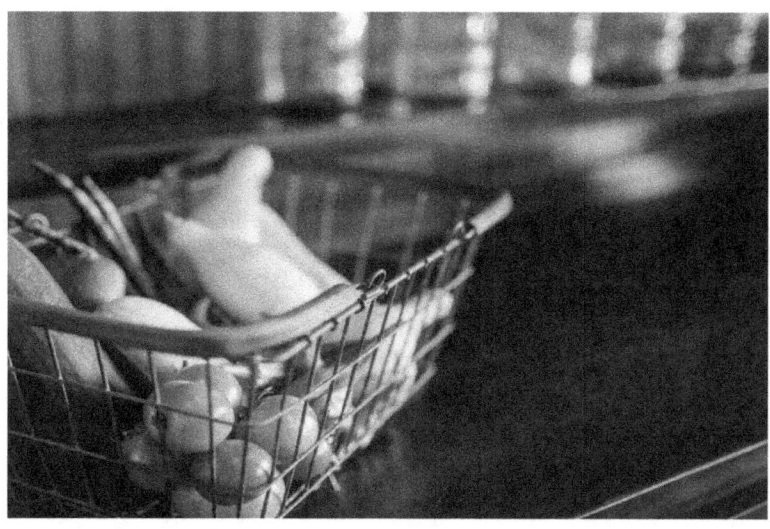

In the day and age of 'superfoods', it can often be difficult to navigate the vast amount of information available. However, one thing is certain – healthy and nutritious food can taste great! In this series of cookbooks, I will showcase recipes featuring healthy and nutritious foods. The recipes in this book are designed to be easily prepared and enjoyed with ingredients that are nutritious, simple, and easily available.

Kale is the focus of this series of recipes. Kale is known for its nutritious profile, including Vitamin A, C and K, fiber and antioxidants. Kale can be a healthy addition to your lifestyle.

Kale comes in many varieties that may be available to you in your local grocery store. The most common form is referred to as a 'bunch' and is on thick green woody stems. For this type of kale, remove the woody stems (as they don't cook well). Then simply wash and use the leaves. If the taste of this kale is too strong, try blanching the kale in hot water or use it in a dish where it is cooked and the flavor profile will become mellow. These bunches come in green and purple varieties, green being the more common variety. Baby kale is another form, and often comes in salad containers. This type of kale does not require you to remove the stems, as they are quite small and soft. This type is idea for salads, and is much more mild in flavor than large leafy kale.

The recipes in this book feature kale as a key ingredient. Some recipes call for more than others. Feel free to use more or less, as is your preference. Some will find kale to have a slightly bitter edge, this can be removed through cooking. If the flavor of kale is snot to your liking, try it in smaller quantities and build up. In each of the recipes, use the type of kale you prefer.

Lastly: organic or nonorganic? Many have asked if kale is something that should be purchased organic. Kale is known to be heavily sprayed with pesticides. If this is a concern to you, then perhaps purchasing organic may be of importance. In either case, as with all produce, make sure to wash well before using

Chapter 1: SMOOTHIES

The following are 5 energizing and healthy, nutrient packed smoothie recipes. The following recipes have been designed with ingredients that are packed full of nutrients, vitamins and fiber and do not use any artificial sweeteners or processed ingredients such as fruit juices (which can often be void of fiber).

Feel free to add more or less of an ingredient you prefer. For the fruit, use fresh or frozen, whichever you have on hand. Frozen fruit will give a creamier and thicker finish to the smoothie compared to fresh.

1. Pineapple and Kale Smoothie

1 cup almond milk

½ fresh or frozen banana

½ cup fresh or frozen pineapple

1 cup packed kale leaves

Place all ingredients in a blender and blend on high until smooth.

2. Strawberry and Kale Smoothie

1 cup almond milk

1 cup fresh or frozen strawberries

1 cup packed kale

1 tablespoon chia seeds

Place the almond milk and chia seeds in the blender and blend on high for 30 seconds. Add the strawberries and kale and blend on high until smooth.

3. Coconut and Kale Smoothie

1 cup coconut milk

1 cup packed kale leaves

½ fresh or frozen banana

honey to taste, optional

Place all ingredients in a blender on high until smooth.

Note: you can use either canned coconut milk or coconut milk from a carton – the canned variety usually contains more coconut fat and will result in a creamier smoothie.

4. Green Avocado Kale Smoothie

1 cup almond milk

½ avocado

1 cup packed kale leaves

1 teaspoon chia seeds

honey to taste, optional

Place all ingredients in a blender until smooth

5. Orange Kale Smoothie

1 cup almond milk

1 orange, peeled, no seeds

1 cup packed kale leaves

1 teaspoon chia seeds

¼ inch slice of fresh ginger, to taste

Place all ingredients in a blender on high until smooth.

Chapter 2: APPETIZERS

Looking for healthier options for your next get together? Or looking for a quick recipe for a night in? The following recipes take classic appetizers and reinvent them to include kale.

1. Kale, Spinach, and Artichoke Dip

Here is a kale packed spin on a traditional appetizer.

8oz cream cheese, room temperature

½ cup mayonnaise

12oz canned artichoke hearts, drained and chopped

½ cup frozen spinach, thawed and drained

4 cups packed chopped kale leaves

2 cloves garlic, minced

½ small red onion, finely diced

½ cup grated Parmesan cheese, divided

¼ cup grated Romano cheese

¼ cup grated Mozzarella cheese

salt and pepper to taste

basil, to taste, optional (3-5 leaves fresh or ½ tbsp dried)

Preheat oven 350 degrees F (175 degrees C).

With a hand held mixer or a stand mixer, mix the cream cheese and mayonnaise until smooth. Add in the rest of the ingredients into the cream cheese and mayonnaise mixture and mix to incorporate well. It may appear that there is too much kale, but it will all cook down.

Place in a baking dish and top with remaining Parmesan cheese. Bake for 25 minutes until bubbly.

2. Kale and Sweet Potato Patties with Paprika Mayo

This recipe packs nutrients and fiber from both the kale and sweet potatoes. Serve this as an appetizer or a side dish. If there are leftovers, they will make for a great lunch.

2 large sweet potatoes

½ bunch kale, ribs removed and chopped

1 egg, beaten

½ cup mayonnaise

½ cup flat leaf parsley

juice and zest of 1 lemon

1 tsp paprika

salt and pepper, to taste

olive oil for pan

In a bowl, add mayonnaise, juice and zest of one lemon, and paprika. Mix well.

In a large pot, place sweet potatoes and cover with cold water and boil on high for 20-30 minutes until soft. Remove, drain and let cool. Once cooled, remove skins.

In a large mixing bowl, place the peeled sweet potatoes and roughly mash. Add in the chopped kale, egg, parsley, salt and pepper. Mix thoroughly until incorporated.

In a skillet on medium high heat, add 1 tablespoon of olive oil. Form patties of the sweet potato and kale mixture and cook until golden brown on each side, approx. 3-5 minutes per side.

These can be kept warm in the oven until ready to serve.

3. Kale Crisps

For the kale lovers out there, here is a recipe that highlights the flavor of kale with a different texture. Instead of reaching for a bag of chips, give these crunchy kale chips a try!

1 bunch kale, stems removed and cut into large pieces
olive oil
½ teaspoon salt

Preheat the oven to 300 degrees F. Line 2 baking trays with parchment paper.

In a bowl, drizzle olive oil over the kale leaves. Using your hands, rub the kale leaves with the olive oil. Add salt and combine.

Arrange the kale leaves on the two trays. Bake in the oven for 10 minutes. Switch the trays and bake for an additional 10-12 minutes. Watch to make sure the kale leaves do not burn.

*Try other seasonings you prefer such as paprika, parmesan cheese, or curry powder.

CHAPTER 3: SALADS

This section highlights kale as the star ingredient for salads. These salads are great as a side and are hearty enough to pair with protein for a great meal. Since kale leaves are more robust than other salad greens, the salads will stay in the fridge for 2-3 days even when dressed. Leftovers will make for a great lunch.

1. Sautéed Kale and Lemon Salad

1 bunch kale, ribs removed and torn into large pieces

1 clove garlic, chopped

juice and zest of one lemon

salt and pepper to taste

1 tablespoon olive oil

In a large skillet, heat to medium high heat. Once heated, all olive oil, kale and garlic. Sautee for 3-5 minutes, until the kale is bright green and slightly wilted and the garlic is fragrant.

Remove the garlic and kale, and place in a large salad bowl. Add juice and zest of lemon, and salt and pepper to taste. Toss the mixture.

Can be served warm or cold.

2. Kale and Roasted Beets

1 bunch kale, ribs removed and torn into bite size pieces

2 beets, stems removed

1 small red onion, sliced lengthwise

4oz goat cheese

2 tablespoons lemon juice

2 tablespoons olive oil

1 tablespoon balsamic vinegar

1 teaspoon honey, optional

salt and pepper to taste

Preheat the oven to 350 degrees F (175 degrees C).

In a small bowl, place 2 tablespoons lemon juice with the onions and allow mixture to sit while you prepare the rest of the salad.

Wrap beets in tin foil and place on a baking tray. Bake in oven for 40 minutes. Let cool before handling. Once cooled, unwrap and remove skins. The skins should come off easily by rubbing the skins away. Cut the beets into bite sized cubes.

For the salad dressing, whisk together olive oil, balsamic vinegar, and honey (if using). Add salt and pepper.

In a large bowl, add the kale leaves, beets, and drained onions. Add the dressing and toss. Add crumbled goat cheese and gently toss.

3. Kale and Orange Salad with Candied Walnuts

1 bunch kale, stems removed, torn into bite size pieces
1 orange, segmented
½ cup walnuts, chopped
2 tablespoons butter
2 tablespoons sugar
2 tablespoons olive oil
1 tablespoon balsamic vinegar
salt and pepper to taste

Heat a large skillet to medium heat. Add butter, sugar and walnuts. Heat gently and allow the mixture to bubble, approx. 5-7 minutes. The walnuts will become toasty, however, keep an eye on them and do not let the walnuts burn. The mixture will take on a golden brown color.

Transfer onto a baking tray lined with parchment and let cool. If they stick together, break the pieces apart.

For the dressing, whisk together olive oil, balsamic vinegar, salt and pepper.

In a large bowl, combine the kale leaves, orange segments, walnuts and dressing. Toss to incorporate.

4. Kale and Quinoa Salad

1 bunch kale, stems removed and chopped

1 cup uncooked quinoa

1/3 dry cranberries

1/3 cup slivered or sliced almonds

2 tablespoons olive oil

1 tablespoon lemon juice

salt and pepper to taste

Cook quinoa according to direction on package. In the last 2-3 minutes of cooking, add in the kale.

Whisk together olive oil, lemon juice, salt and pepper.

Once the quinoa has finished cooking, add the cranberries, almonds and olive oil mixture. Serve warm or refrigerate and serve cold.

5. Kale Caesar Salad

1 bunch kale leaves, stems removed and torn into bite size pieces

1 package croutons

bacon bits, premade or homemade, to preference

½ cup olive oil

juice and zest of 1 lemon

1 teaspoon anchovy paste

2 cloves garlic, grated

1 teaspoon Dijon mustard

1 teaspoon Worcestershire sauce

black pepper, to taste

¼ cup parmesan cheese

Whisk together olive oil, juice and zest of lemon, anchovy paste, Dijon mustard, garlic, and pepper. Add parmesan cheese.

In a salad bowl, toss kale leaves with salad dressing. Add croutons and bacon bits. Add more parmesan cheese if desired.

6. Kale and Radish Salad

1 bunch kale leaves, stems removed and torn into bite size pieces

1 cup radish, sliced

1 quart cherry tomatoes

¼ cup olive oil

2 tablespoons balsamic vinegar

1 teaspoon honey

salt and pepper to taste

2 tbsp sunflower seeds, optional

Whisk together olive oil, balsamic vinegar, honey, salt and pepper.

In a large bowl, add kale leaves, radishes and tomatoes. Add salad dressing and toss. Top with sunflower seeds, if using.

Chapter 4: MAINS

These next 6 recipes bring kale to the dinner table as one of the main ingredients. As always, use as little or as much kale as you prefer.

1. Chicken with Kale and Brussel Sprouts

1 lb chicken thighs, cut into 1 inch cubes

1 bunch kale leaves, stems removed and roughly chopped

2 lbs brussel sprouts, halved

1 small onion, chopped

3 cloves garlic

1 teaspoon chili flakes

½ cup chicken stock

olive oil

In a large skillet, heat to medium high and add olive oil and chicken, browning on all sides. Be careful not to over crowd the pan (do this step in batches if necessary). Transfer cooked chicken to a plate lined with paper towel.

In a large skillet heat to medium high and add olive oil, brussle sprouts and onions. Cook until brussel sprouts are golden and appear caramelized, approx. 10 minutes. Add chili flakes, garlic and kale. Cook for another 1-2 minutes.

Add chicken stock deglaze pan. Add chicken and heat mixture through.

Serve with brown rice, or another grain, for a complete meal.

2. Tuscan kale and sausage pasta

6 oz penne, or other small pasta

1 lb sausage of choice, casing removed and coarsely chopped

1/2 cup sundried tomatoes in oil, drained and chopped

1 full bunch kale, ribs removed, and chopped

2 tablespoons olive oil

2 cloves garlic, grated

1 small onion, chopped

1/2 cup heavy cream

1/2 cup dry white wine, or substitute with chicken stock

1/2 cup flat leaf parsley, chopped

1/2 cup grated Parmesan cheese

Salt and pepper to taste

1 teaspoon chili flakes, or to taste

Cook pasta as per direction on the box. Reserve 1 cup of the starchy water for the sauce.

Heat a large pan on medium-high heat. Once heated add olive oil and onions and sautée for 2-3 min, until soft and translucent. Add garlic and sautée for an additional 30 seconds. Add the sausage, sundried tomatoes and chilli flakes and cook until sausage has cooked through and slightly browned, 4-5 minutes. Add white wine (or chicken stock) and deglaze the pan (scrape off all the brown bits on the pan, this is flavor). Add salt and pepper. Simmer until wine has evaporated, 3-5 minutes. Add cream and kale to the pan.

Add the cooked and drained pasta to the pan and mix. If the sauce appears to thick, add the reserved starchy cooking water from the pasta to thin out the sauce to the desired consistency.

Add Parmesan cheese and parsley, and mix into the pasta.

Serve hot.

3. Kale and Pork Tortellini

1 large package tortellini

1 lb ground pork

1 bunch kale leave, stems removed and chopped

1 small onion, diced

4 cloves garlic, chopped

2 teaspoons chili flakes

½ cup chopped parsley

¼ cup chopped basil

1-2 tablespoons cream cheese, optional

¼ cup olive oil

salt and pepper to taste

Cook tortellini according to package directions. Reserve 1 cup of the starchy cooking water for the sauce.

In a large skillet on medium high heat, add olive oil, ground pork, onion, garlic and chili flakes. Cook until pork in cooked through and slightly browned. Add the kale leaves and cook until wilted, 1-2 minutes. Add salt and pepper.

Add 1-2 tablespoons of the starchy cooking water to the sauce to deglaze the pan. If using cream cheese, add in here.

Add pasta, parsley and basil. Toss to combine.

Serve hot.

4. Kale and Chorizo Slow Cooker Stew

1 bunch kale leaves, stems removed, chopped

1 lb chorizo sausage, casing removed and chopped

1 lb mushrooms, sliced

1 small onion, chopped

1 carrot, diced

1 celery stalk, diced

1 teaspoon chili flakes or crushed red chili powder

2 cloves garlic

6 cups chicken stock

2 tablespoon olive oil, divided

salt and pepper to taste

In a skillet on medium high heat, add olive oil, onion, celery, carrot, and garlic. Cook for 3-5 minutes, until soft. Transfer to slow cooker.

In the same skillet, add olive oil and cook chorizo sausage until browned. Transfer to slow cooker.

In the slow cooker, add chicken stock, mushrooms, chili flakes/red chili powder, salt and pepper. Cook on med-high for 4-6 hours.

In the last 30 minutes, add the kale.

Serve hot.

5. Tortellini and Kale Soup

1 small package tortellini

1 bunch kale leaves, stems removed and chopped

6 cups chicken stock

1 small onion, chopped

1 carrot, diced

1 celery stalk, diced

1 teaspoon chili flakes or crushed red chili powder

1 cloves garlic

6 cups chicken stock

1 tablespoon olive oil

salt and pepper to taste

In a large pot on medium high heat, add olive oil, onion, carrot, and celery. Cook until soft, approx. 5-7 minutes. Add garlic, chili flakes/chili powder, salt and pepper.

Add in chicken stock and bring to boil. Add in tortellini and cook according to time on package. Add kale in the last one minute of cooking.

Serve hot.

6. Mushroom and Kale Risotto

1lb mushrooms, chopped

½ bunch kale leaves, stems removed, finely chopped

½ small white onion, chopped

1 clove garlic

1 cup dry white wine

salt and pepper to taste

1 cup Arborio rice

6 cups chicken stock, warmed

½ cup parmesan cheese

2 tablespoons butter

2 tablespoons olive oil

1 teaspoon hot paprika

In a large pot on medium high heat, add olive oil and mushrooms. Cook for 7-10minutes, until slightly browned. Add onion, garlic, salt, pepper and hot paprika (if using).

Cook an additional 4-5 minutes. Add dry white wine. Cook until the wine has evaporated.

Add in 1 cup Arborio rice. Add in ½ cup warmed chicken stock and stir until the stock is absorbed. Continue adding ½ cup of the chicken stock at a time until all the stock has been used.

Add in the Parmesan cheese and butter and stir.

7. Linguini with Kale Pesto

1 lb linguini

1 bunch kale leaves, stems removed

1 cup olive oil

1 cup chopped basil

½ cup walnuts

½ cup parmesan cheese

2 cloves garlic

salt and pepper to taste

Cook pasta according to directions on package. Reserve ½ cup of the starchy cooking water.

In a food processor add in kale, basil, garlic, walnuts and cheese. Once the food processer is on, drizzle in the olive oil. For a thinner pesto, add in extra olive oil.

In a large bowl, add the linguini and a few tablespoons of the pesto until the desired amount is reached. Use 1-2 tablespoons of the starchy cooking water to create a sauce.

The pesto can be stored in the refrigerator for up to 2 weeks, or kept frozen for up to 6 months.

*Tip: Freeze in an ice cube tray for quick and easy use. Pesto can be used to marinate meats and vegetables as well.

CONCLUSION

Thank you again for purchasing this book!

I hope this book was able to help you to find Kale recipes that you can use every day with ingredients you have at home. It is something I am passionate about and have adopted into my life style. It takes time and effort but has lead to me being more healthy and to feel great! I hope this helps you with your life and please let me know about how this book has helped you.

The next step is to stay vigilant and maintain your newly realized lifestyle.

Finally, if you enjoyed this book, then I'd like to ask you for a favor, would you be kind enough to leave a review for this book on Amazon? It'd be greatly appreciated!

Thank you and good luck!

The information herein is offered for informational purposes solely, and is universal as so. The presentation of the information is without contract or any type of guarantee assurance.

The trademarks that are used are without any consent, and the publication of the trademark is without permission or backing by the trademark owner. All trademarks and brands within this book are for clarifying purposes only and are the owned by the owners themselves, not affiliated with this document.

www.ingramcontent.com/pod-product-compliance
Lightning Source LLC
Chambersburg PA
CBHW072026280526
45788CB00007B/2693